Diabetes and Life

A Journey of Management, Faith, and Healing

Alison Spence

Copyright © *Alison Spence*, 2025

All Rights Reserved

This book is subject to the condition that no part of this book is to be reproduced, transmitted in any form or means; electronic or mechanical, stored in a retrieval system, photocopied, recorded, scanned, or otherwise. Any of these actions require the proper written permission of the author.

Table of Contents

Chapter 1 Understanding Diabetes 1
What is Diabetes? 1
Types of Diabetes 1
Causes and Risk Factors 3
Symptoms and Early Detection 4
The Impact of Diabetes on the Body 4

Chapter 2 The Science behind Blood Sugar 6
How the Body Regulates Glucose 6
The Role of Insulin 6
Hyperglycaemia vs. Hypoglycaemia 7
Long-Term Effects of Poor Blood Sugar Control 7

Chapter 3 Diagnosis and Monitoring 9
Common Tests 9
Continuous Glucose Monitoring (CGM) 9
Self-Monitoring Tips 10
Understanding Your Results 10

Chapter 4 Management through Nutrition 11
The Role of Diet in Diabetes Management 11
Creating a Balanced Meal Plan 11
Glycemic Index (GI) and Its Importance 12
Healthy Alternatives and Snack Ideas 12

Chapter 5 Physical Activity and Diabetes 13
Benefits of Exercise 13
Types of Exercises for Diabetics 13
Tips for Safe Workouts 13
Managing Blood Sugar during Exercise 13

Chapter 6 Medication and Technology 14
Overview of Diabetes Medications 14
Insulin: Types, Dosages, and Administration 14
Emerging Technologies in Diabetes Care 14
Personalized Medicine in Diabetes Management............................15

Chapter 7 Complications and Prevention 16
Common Complications 16
Early Detection and Management 16
Preventive Strategies and Lifestyle Adjustments.............................16

Chapter 8 Living Well with Diabetes 18
Traveling with Diabetes 18
Managing Diabetes in Special Situations 18
Healthy Aging with Diabetes...19
Finding Joy and Balance in Everyday Life 19

Chapter 9 God's Creation, Sin, and Death: A Biblical Perspective 21
Creation of Man and God's Design of the Body............................21
The Introduction of Sin and Its Impact on Health (Genesis 3) 21
The fall and the Origin of Suffering and Death 21
Redemption and Hope through Christ..21
Integrating Faith in Managing Chronic Conditions........................21

Chapter 10 Faith and Healing in Diabetes Management............ 22
The Role of Prayer and Faith in Healing...22
Finding Strength in Scripture during Health Struggles 22
Practical Steps to Trust God in Your Diabetes Journey..................22
Stories of Faith and Resilience from Diabetics 22

Chapter 11 The Future of Diabetes Management 24
Advances in Research and Treatment..24
The Promise of Gene Therapy 24
Artificial Pancreas Technology...24

The Vision for a Diabetes-Free Future 24

Chapter 12 Resources and Tools 25
Recipes for Diabetic-Friendly Meals 25

Templates for Blood Sugar Tracking 25

Recommended Apps and Devices 25

Support Groups and Online Communities 25

Chapter 13 Conclusion: A Journey of Hope and Resilience 26
Recap of Key Concepts 26

Encouragement for the Future 26

Embracing Life Fully Despite Diabetes 26

References 27
Scientific References: 27

Faith-Based References: 28

Patient-Friendly Resources: 28

Chapter 1
Understanding Diabetes

Diabetes is a chronic medical condition that occurs when the body cannot effectively regulate blood sugar (glucose) levels. Glucose is a vital energy source for the body, but when its levels become too high or too low, it can lead to serious health complications. Managing diabetes requires a combination of lifestyle changes, medical intervention, and ongoing monitoring.

What is Diabetes?

Diabetes is characterized by elevated levels of glucose in the blood due to the body's inability to produce enough insulin or to use insulin effectively. Insulin, a hormone produced by the pancreas, helps move glucose from the bloodstream into cells, where it is used for energy. When this process is disrupted, glucose builds up in the blood, leading to hyperglycaemia (high blood sugar). Over time, uncontrolled hyperglycaemia can damage vital organs and systems, including the heart, kidneys, eyes, and nerves.

Types of Diabetes

1. **Type 1 Diabetes:**
    - **Definition:** An autoimmune condition where the immune system attacks insulin-producing beta cells in the pancreas. As a result, the body produces little or no insulin.
    - **Key Features:**
        - Often diagnosed in children and young adults, though it can occur at any age.
        - Requires lifelong insulin therapy.

- **Causes:** The exact cause is unknown, but genetic predisposition and environmental triggers are believed to play a role.

2. **Type 2 Diabetes:**
   - **Definition:** A metabolic disorder where the body becomes resistant to insulin, and the pancreas cannot produce enough insulin to compensate.
   - **Key Features:**
     - Most common type of diabetes, typically developing in adults but increasingly seen in children.
     - Often linked to lifestyle factors such as poor diet, lack of exercise, and obesity.
   - **Causes:** Genetic factors, obesity, physical inactivity, and other lifestyle factors.

3. **Gestational Diabetes:**
   - **Definition:** A form of diabetes that develops during pregnancy and usually resolves after childbirth.
   - **Key Features:**
     - Increases the risk of complications for both mother and baby.
     - Women with gestational diabetes are at higher risk of developing Type 2 diabetes later in life.
   - **Causes:** Hormonal changes during pregnancy that affect insulin sensitivity.

4. **Other Forms of Diabetes:**
   - **Monogenic Diabetes:** Caused by a single gene mutation (e.g., MODY - Maturity Onset Diabetes of the Young).

- o **Secondary Diabetes:** Resulting from other medical conditions or medications, such as pancreatitis or steroid use.

Causes and Risk Factors

Causes of Diabetes:

- **Type 1 Diabetes:** Autoimmune destruction of insulin-producing cells.
- **Type 2 Diabetes:** Insulin resistance and beta-cell dysfunction.
- **Gestational Diabetes:** Hormonal changes during pregnancy leading to insulin resistance.

Risk Factors:

1. **Type 1 Diabetes:**
    - o Family history of autoimmune diseases.
    - o Environmental triggers, such as viral infections.

2. **Type 2 Diabetes:**
    - o Obesity and physical inactivity.
    - o Family history of diabetes.
    - o Age over 45 years.
    - o Ethnic background (higher prevalence in certain groups, e.g., South Asians, African-Americans).
    - o Conditions like polycystic ovary syndrome (PCOS) and hypertension.

3. **Gestational Diabetes:**
    - o Previous history of gestational diabetes.
    - o Being overweight before pregnancy.

- Advanced maternal age.

Symptoms and Early Detection

Common Symptoms of Diabetes:

- Increased thirst and frequent urination.
- Unexplained weight loss.
- Fatigue and weakness.
- Blurred vision.
- Slow-healing wounds and frequent infections.
- Tingling or numbness in hands and feet (in Type 2 Diabetes).

Early Detection:

- Regular screening for individuals with risk factors.
- Routine blood tests such as fasting blood sugar, HbA1c, or oral glucose tolerance tests (OGTT).
- Awareness of prediabetes symptoms like mild fatigue or weight gain.

The Impact of Diabetes on the Body

Uncontrolled diabetes can affect various organs and systems in the body, leading to both acute and chronic complications.

1. **Cardiovascular System:**
   - Increases the risk of heart disease, stroke, and hypertension.//
2. **Kidneys:**
   - Can lead to diabetic nephropathy (kidney damage), eventually requiring dialysis.

3. **Eyes:**
   - May cause diabetic retinopathy, cataracts, or glaucoma, potentially leading to blindness.
4. **Nerves:**
   - Results in diabetic neuropathy, causing pain, tingling, or numbness, especially in the feet.
5. **Immune System:**
   - Impairs wound healing and increases susceptibility to infections.

Managing diabetes effectively can significantly reduce the risk of these complications, highlighting the importance of early detection and ongoing care.

This foundational understanding of diabetes lays the groundwork for exploring its management strategies and the integration of faith and resilience in the journey toward better health.

Chapter 2
The Science behind Blood Sugar

Glucose, a simple sugar derived from the foods we eat, is the body's primary source of energy. Maintaining blood sugar levels within a healthy range is essential for optimal functioning of the body. This chapter delves into how the body regulates glucose, the role of insulin, and the effects of imbalances in blood sugar.

How the Body Regulates Glucose

The body maintains blood sugar levels through a dynamic balance involving:

1. **Food Intake:** Glucose enters the bloodstream after digestion, primarily from carbohydrates.
2. **Hormonal Regulation:** Insulin and glucagon, hormones produced by the pancreas, play pivotal roles in maintaining balance.
3. **Storage and Release:**
    - Excess glucose is stored as glycogen in the liver and muscles.
    - During fasting or physical activity, stored glycogen is broken down to maintain energy levels.

The Role of Insulin

Insulin, produced by the beta cells in the pancreas, acts as a "key" that allows glucose to enter cells for energy. It performs several functions:

1. **Facilitates Glucose Uptake:** Helps muscles, fat, and other tissues absorb glucose.

2. **Promotes Storage:** Encourages the liver to store excess glucose as glycogen.
3. **Regulates Fat and Protein Metabolism:** Ensures that glucose is the primary energy source, sparing proteins and fats.

Hyperglycaemia vs. Hypoglycaemia

1. **Hyperglycaemia (High Blood Sugar):**
   - **Causes:** Insufficient insulin, insulin resistance, overeating, stress, or illness.
   - **Symptoms:** Thirst, frequent urination, fatigue, blurred vision.
   - **Risks:** Prolonged hyperglycaemia can lead to complications like neuropathy, nephropathy, and cardiovascular disease.
2. **Hypoglycaemia (Low Blood Sugar):**
   - **Causes:** Overdose of insulin or medications, skipping meals, excessive exercise.
   - **Symptoms:** Dizziness, sweating, shaking, confusion, or even loss of consciousness.
   - **Risks:** Severe hypoglycaemia can result in seizures, coma, or death if untreated.

Long-Term Effects of Poor Blood Sugar Control

Uncontrolled blood sugar levels over time can cause:

1. **Microvascular Complications:**
   - **Retinopathy:** Damage to the blood vessels in the eyes, leading to vision problems.
   - **Nephropathy:** Kidney damage, potentially resulting in dialysis.

- **Neuropathy:** Nerve damage causing pain, tingling, or numbness.

2. **Microvascular Complications:**
    - **Cardiovascular Disease:** Increased risk of heart attack, stroke, and atherosclerosis.

3. **Other Effects:**
    - Reduced immunity, delayed wound healing, and increased risk of infections.

Chapter 3
Diagnosis and Monitoring

Accurate diagnosis and regular monitoring are essential for effective diabetes management.

Common Tests

1. **HbA1c (Glycated Haemoglobin Test):**
    - Reflects average blood sugar levels over the past 2-3 months.
    - Normal: Below 5.7%; Prediabetes: 5.7%-6.4%; Diabetes: 6.5% or higher.

2. **Fasting Blood Sugar (FBS):**
    - Measures blood sugar after an overnight fast.
    - Normal: Below 100 mg/dL; Prediabetes: 100-125 mg/dL; Diabetes: 126 mg/dL or higher.

3. **Oral Glucose Tolerance Test (OGTT):**
    - Measures blood sugar 2 hours after consuming a glucose drink.
    - Normal: Below 140 mg/dL; Prediabetes: 140-199 mg/dL; Diabetes: 200 mg/dL or higher.

Continuous Glucose Monitoring (CGM)

- CGMs use sensors to provide real-time blood sugar readings throughout the day.
- Helps identify trends and patterns in blood sugar levels.
- Useful for individuals on intensive insulin therapy or experiencing frequent hypo- or hyperglycaemia.

Self-Monitoring Tips

1. **Frequency of Monitoring:**
   - Type 1 Diabetes: Multiple checks daily.
   - Type 2 Diabetes: Based on the treatment plan, typically before meals and at bedtime.
2. **Technique:**
   - Use clean hands and the side of a fingertip for testing.
   - Keep a log of results to share with healthcare providers.
3. **Post-Meal Testing:**
   - Check 1-2 hours after eating to assess the impact of meals on blood sugar.

Understanding Your Results

1. **Target Blood Sugar Ranges:**
   - Fasting: 80-130 mg/dL.
   - 2 Hours Post-Meal: Less than 180 mg/dL.
2. **Interpreting Trends:**
   - Look for consistent patterns of high or low readings.
   - Adjust diet, medication, or activity levels accordingly with guidance from a healthcare provider.
3. **Communicating with Your Doctor:**
   - Share logs, CGM data, and any symptoms to optimize treatment plans.

Proper understanding of blood sugar regulation, diagnostic tools, and monitoring techniques empowers individuals to take control of their diabetes journey, ensuring better long-term health outcomes.

Chapter 4
Management through Nutrition

The Role of Diet in Diabetes Management

Diet plays a central role in diabetes care. Proper nutrition helps:

- Maintain steady blood sugar levels.
- Reduce the risk of complications.
- Support overall health and well-being.

The goal is to consume nutrient-dense foods in appropriate portions, ensuring a balance of carbohydrates, proteins, and healthy fats.

Creating a Balanced Meal Plan

1. **Portion Control:** Use the plate method:
   - Half the plate: Non-starchy vegetables (e.g., spinach, broccoli).
   - One-quarter: Lean proteins (e.g., chicken, fish, tofu).
   - One-quarter: Whole grains or starchy vegetables (e.g., quinoa, sweet potatoes).

2. **Carbohydrate Counting:**
   - Monitor carb intake to prevent spikes in blood sugar.
   - Choose complex carbs like whole grains, legumes, and vegetables.

3. **Meal Timing:**
   - Eat at consistent times to avoid blood sugar fluctuations.
   - Include healthy snacks if meals are spaced far apart.

Glycemic Index (GI) and Its Importance

- **Definition:** GI measures how quickly foods raise blood sugar levels.
- **Low-GI Foods (Best Choice):**
    - Examples: Lentils, oats, nuts, and most vegetables.
    - Provide a slow, steady release of glucose.
- **High-GI Foods (Limit):**
    - Examples: White bread, sugary snacks, and processed cereals.
    - Cause rapid blood sugar spikes.

Healthy Alternatives and Snack Ideas

1. **Healthy Swaps:**
    - White rice → Quinoa or brown rice.
    - Sugary drinks → Water with lemon or herbal teas.
    - Chips → Air-popped popcorn or roasted chickpeas.
2. **Snack Ideas:**
    - A handful of nuts or seeds.
    - Greek yogurt with berries.
    - Sliced veggies with hummus.

Chapter 5
Physical Activity and Diabetes

Benefits of Exercise

- Improves insulin sensitivity.
- Helps with weight management.
- Reduces the risk of cardiovascular complications.
- Enhances overall mental and physical well-being.

Types of Exercises for Diabetics

1. **Aerobic Exercises:** Walking, swimming, or cycling.
2. **Strength Training:** Resistance bands, light weights.
3. **Flexibility and Balance:** Yoga, stretching, tai chi.

Tips for Safe Workouts

- Check blood sugar before and after exercise.
- Stay hydrated during workouts.
- Always carry a fast-acting carbohydrate (e.g., glucose tablets) in case of hypoglycaemia.

Managing Blood Sugar during Exercise

- Monitor patterns to adjust insulin or carb intake.
- Avoid exercise during peak insulin activity to prevent lows.
- Consult a healthcare provider for tailored exercise plans.

Chapter 6
Medication and Technology

Overview of Diabetes Medications

1. **Oral Medications:**
    - **Metformin:** Reduces glucose production in the liver.
    - **SGLT2 Inhibitors:** Promote glucose excretion via urine.
    - **DPP-4 Inhibitors:** Increase insulin release post-meal.
2. **Injectable Medications:**
    - GLP-1 receptor agonists (e.g., liraglutide) to slow digestion and enhance insulin release.

Insulin: Types, Dosages, and Administration

1. **Types of Insulin:**
    - Rapid-acting: Taken with meals.
    - Long-acting: Provides basal insulin throughout the day.
2. **Administration Tips:**
    - Rotate injection sites to avoid scarring.
    - Use insulin pens or pumps for convenience.

Emerging Technologies in Diabetes Care

- **Insulin Pumps:** Deliver precise insulin doses automatically.
- **Continuous Glucose Monitors (CGMs):** Provide real-time glucose readings, reducing the need for frequent fingersticks.

Personalized Medicine in Diabetes Management

- Tailored treatment plans based on genetics, lifestyle, and glucose patterns.
- Future advancements in artificial pancreas technology.

Chapter 7
Complications and Prevention

Common Complications

1. **Neuropathy:** Nerve damage leading to pain or numbness.
2. **Retinopathy:** Eye damage that can cause vision loss.
3. **Nephropathy:** Kidney damage that may progress to failure.

Early Detection and Management

- Regular screenings for complications:
    - Annual eye exams for retinopathy.
    - Kidney function tests (e.g., microalbuminuria).
    - Foot checks for ulcers or infections.
- Immediate intervention for any detected abnormalities.

Preventive Strategies and Lifestyle Adjustments

1. **Blood Sugar Control:**
    - Maintain HbA1c levels within the target range.
2. **Blood Pressure and Cholesterol:**
    - Manage with diet, exercise, and medications if needed.
3. **Lifestyle Adjustments:**
    - Avoid smoking and limit alcohol intake.
    - Stay active and maintain a healthy weight.

This comprehensive section integrates practical advice and modern advancements to empower readers in managing diabetes effectively while preventing complications.

Chapter 8
Living Well with Diabetes

Traveling with Diabetes

Traveling with diabetes requires planning, but it shouldn't stop you from exploring the world. Here are practical tips to ensure a smooth journey:

1. **Pre-Trip Preparations:**
    - Visit your healthcare provider to discuss travel plans.
    - Pack enough medication and supplies for the trip, plus extras.
    - Carry a letter from your doctor explaining your condition and medications.

2. **During Travel:**
    - Keep medication in your carry-on bag to avoid exposure to extreme temperatures.
    - Maintain meal schedules, especially during long flights or time zone changes.
    - Stay hydrated and stretch during travel to reduce the risk of blood clots.

3. **Emergency Preparedness:**
    - Wear a medical ID bracelet indicating you have diabetes.
    - Know the locations of nearby medical facilities.

Managing Diabetes in Special Situations

1. **Sick Days:**
    - Monitor blood sugar more frequently as illness can cause fluctuations.

- Stay hydrated and consume easily digestible foods if appetite decreases.
- Continue taking medications unless advised otherwise by a doctor.

2. **Surgery:**
   - Discuss your condition with the surgical team beforehand.
   - Ensure your blood sugar levels are stable pre-surgery.
   - Post-surgery, monitor closely as healing can impact glucose control.

Healthy Aging with Diabetes

Aging with diabetes presents unique challenges but can be managed effectively:

1. **Focus on Preventing Complications:**
   - Regular eye exams, kidney tests, and foot checks.
   - Address cardiovascular risks with lifestyle adjustments.

2. **Stay Active:**
   - Engage in gentle exercises like walking or tai chi to improve circulation and mobility.

3. **Simplify Management:**
   - Use tools like pill organizers or apps to keep track of medications and appointments.

Finding Joy and Balance in Everyday Life

Living with diabetes involves more than managing blood sugar—it's about embracing life fully:

1. **Practice Gratitude:** Focus on the positives in your life.

2. **Pursue Hobbies:** Engage in activities that bring you joy and fulfilment.
3. **Build Relationships:** Lean on friends and family for emotional support.

Chapter 9
God's Creation, Sin, and Death: A Biblical Perspective

Creation of Man and God's Design of the Body

God designed the human body with incredible complexity and resilience, reflecting His creativity and wisdom (Psalm 139:14).

The Introduction of Sin and Its Impact on Health (Genesis 3)

Sin entered the world through Adam and Eve's disobedience, bringing suffering, sickness, and death. This separation from God disrupted the harmony of creation.

The fall and the Origin of Suffering and Death

The fall led to physical and spiritual death, making humanity susceptible to diseases, including chronic conditions like diabetes.

Redemption and Hope through Christ

Through Jesus Christ, redemption and healing are possible. Believers can find hope and strength in God's promise of eternal life and restoration (John 3:16).

Integrating Faith in Managing Chronic Conditions

Faith provides a foundation for resilience, helping individuals cope with the challenges of chronic illness through prayer, trust in God, and community support.

Chapter 10
Faith and Healing in Diabetes Management

The Role of Prayer and Faith in Healing

Prayer can bring peace and comfort, even when physical healing isn't immediate. Trusting God's plan helps maintain hope and courage.

Finding Strength in Scripture during Health Struggles

Verses like Philippians 4:13 ("I can do all things through Christ who strengthens me") remind us that God's strength is always available.

Practical Steps to Trust God in Your Diabetes Journey

- Begin each day with prayer and reflection.
- Seek a supportive faith community for encouragement.
- Trust in God's guidance for decisions about your health.

Stories of Faith and Resilience from Diabetics

A Story of Hope, Faith, and Healing

For 43 years, my mother has lived with diabetes—a journey filled with challenges, adjustments, and moments of uncertainty. Yet, through it all, her unwavering **faith in God** has been her foundation, her source of strength, and her beacon of hope.

From the beginning of her diagnosis, my mother chose to place her trust in God, believing that He would guide her through every step of managing her health. She embraced the recommended lifestyle and diet advice, finding inspiration in the principles outlined in the Bible—principles that emphasize **balance, moderation, and care for the body as God's temple** (1 Corinthians 6:19-20).

Her faith-filled approach to managing diabetes has been a testimony to us all. She has shown us how to combine practical wisdom with spiritual trust, making prayer a daily part of her health routine and leaning on Scriptures like **Psalm 46:1**: *"God is our refuge and strength, an ever-present help in trouble."*

Even on the hard days—when her energy was low, or her blood sugar levels were challenging to control—her hope never wavered. She reminded us that this life is not the end. Her belief in God's promise of **eternal life through Christ Jesus** has been her ultimate assurance. It has given her—and us—hope that one day, in a future free from sickness and pain, we will experience the joy of living forever (Revelation 21:4).

This faith-filled journey has taught our family the importance of trusting God's plan, even in the face of long-term illness. It has shown us the power of combining faith with action, hope with perseverance, and prayer with practical care.

My mother's story is a beautiful reminder that, even amidst health challenges, there is always **hope**. Through faith, trust in God, and the wisdom to care for ourselves as He intends, we can face each day with confidence and assurance of His promises.

To anyone reading this who might be battling illness or caring for a loved one, know this: **you are not alone**. God walks with you, and His promises bring strength for today and bright hope for tomorrow. Let this story encourage you to trust, to persevere, and to embrace the hope of a future where we will live forever in His presence. ♡

Chapter 11
The Future of Diabetes Management

Advances in Research and Treatment

Ongoing research is improving understanding and treatment options, including medications and personalized care.

The Promise of Gene Therapy

Emerging therapies hold the potential to reverse diabetes at the genetic level, offering hope for a cure.

Artificial Pancreas Technology

Devices that mimic the pancreas's function are becoming more advanced, offering better glucose control and quality of life.

The Vision for a Diabetes-Free Future

With continued progress, a future without diabetes is a realistic goal, providing hope to millions worldwide.

Chapter 12
Resources and Tools

Recipes for Diabetic-Friendly Meals

- Simple, delicious recipes for balanced meals that support blood sugar control.

Templates for Blood Sugar Tracking

- Printable charts or app recommendations to monitor blood sugar trends.

Recommended Apps and Devices

- Apps for meal planning, glucose tracking, and medication reminders.

Support Groups and Online Communities

- Resources to connect with others facing similar challenges.

Chapter 13
Conclusion: A Journey of Hope and Resilience

Recap of Key Concepts

Managing diabetes is about balancing medical care, lifestyle, and emotional well-being.

Encouragement for the Future

Even in the face of challenges, hope, faith, and resilience can lead to a fulfilling life.

Embracing Life Fully Despite Diabetes

By combining faith, science, and a supportive community, individuals can thrive and live abundantly, despite a diabetes diagnosis.

References

Scientific References:

1. **World Health Organization (WHO):**
   - Diabetes Fact Sheets: https://www.who.int

2. **American Diabetes Association (ADA):**
   - Standards of Medical Care in Diabetes: https://diabetes.org

3. **National Institute for Health and Care Excellence (NICE):**
   - Guidelines for Diabetes Management: https://www.nice.org.uk

4. **Centers for Disease Control and Prevention (CDC):**
   - Diabetes Information and Statistics: https://www.cdc.gov

5. **International Diabetes Federation (IDF):**
   - Global Diabetes Reports: https://www.idf.org

6. **Joslin Diabetes Center:**
   - Clinical Care and Research Publications: https://www.joslin.org

7. **Peer-Reviewed Articles:**
   - American Journal of Clinical Nutrition: Studies on dietary impact on diabetes.
   - Lancet Diabetes & Endocrinology: Cutting-edge diabetes research.

8. **Books:**
   - "Diabetes: A Practical Guide to Managing Your Health" by David Levy.
   - "Think Like a Pancreas" by Gary Scheiner.
9. **Technology Resources:**
   - Continuous Glucose Monitoring and Insulin Pump Manufacturers (e.g., Medtronic, Dexcom, Abbott).

Faith-Based References:

1. **The Bible:**
   - Genesis 1–3 (Creation, Sin, and the Fall)
   - Philippians 4:13 (Strength through Christ)
   - John 3:16 (Hope through Redemption)
   - Psalm 139:14 (Fearfully and Wonderfully Made)
2. **Books on Faith and Health:**
   - "The Daniel Plan: 40 Days to a Healthier Life" by Rick Warren, Daniel Amen, and Mark Hyman.
   - "God's Healing Promises" by Charles Spurgeon.
3. **Faith-Based Health Resources:**
   - Christian Medical and Dental Associations: https://www.cmda.org
   - Faith and Diabetes Support Groups (local or online).

Patient-Friendly Resources:

1. **Diabetes UK:** https://www.diabetes.org.uk
   - Practical advice for diabetes management.

2. **MySugr App:** Tools for tracking blood glucose and managing diabetes.

3. **Local Diabetes Associations:**
    - Australian Diabetes Society
    - Diabetes Canada

www.ingramcontent.com/pod-product-compliance
Lightning Source LLC
Chambersburg PA
CBHW061732070526
44583CB00024B/3110